H

PHYSICAL FITN

by

VIKRAM DAMODHAR SATPUTE

TABLE OF CONTENTS

CHAPTER

I

CHAPTER I

INTRODUCTION

1.1 CONCEPTUAL FRAMEWORK

The expert committee of the World Health Organization described physical fitness as the ability to undertake muscular work satisfactorily. Physical fitness is the capacity to early out, reasonably well, various forms of physical activities, without being unduly tired and includes qualities important to the individual's health and well-being. Every person has a different level of physical fitness which may change with time, place of work, situation and there is also an interaction between the daily activities, and the fitness of an individual, the point if where to put the level of optimum fitness. From the physiological point of view physical fitness may say to be ability at the body to adopt and recover from strenuous exercise.

The World Health Organization defines health as: "Health is physical, mental, social and spiritual wellbeing, not merely the absence of disease and infirmity." The focus of health has changed over the years from an emphasis on mainly trying to reduce sickness and death, rather attention has turned more and more to health promotion. Health represents a dynamic state of positive wellbeing where habits that promote health are practiced, lowering the risk of premature disease and death.

Scientists and doctors have known for years that substantial benefits can be gained from regular physical activity (Manley, 1996). Today we have strong evidence to indicate that regular physical activity provides clear and substantial health gains. Physical activity is so directly related to preventing disease and premature death and to maintaining a high quality of life that its importance must be understood at all levels.

It is a known fact that Physical inactivity amongst the population is now wide spread. One out of four adults currently has sedentary lifestyles with no leisure time physical activity (Manley,1996). An additional one-third of adults are insufficiently active to achieve health benefits. The prevalence of inactivity varies by gender, age, ethnicity, health status and geographic region.

In India, children become far less active as they move through adolescence and it is found that obesity is increasing among children. Childhood and adolescence may thus be pivotal times for preventing sedentary behaviour among adults. School based interventions have shown to be successful in increasing physical activity levels (Manley, 1996). Recent newspaper reports have highlighted increasing obesity amongst school going children. Prevention of childhood obesity has the potential of preventing Cardio Vascular Diseases in adults.

Physical activity is directly related to physical fitness. Regular physical activity or cardio respiratory fitness decreases the risk of cardio vascular disease mortality in general and of coronary heart disease mortality in particular (Manley, 1996). Various," Health surveys and development committee Government of India" also found poor status of public health. Several other surveys in the west have clearly pointed out that for optimal health, people of all ages have to be physically active on most days.

According to current thinking, health related Physical fitness is concerned with the development of those qualities that offer protection against disease and frequently are associated with physical activity. For example, certain physiological and psychological factors often affected by physical activity are thought to cause some degenerative disease. Thus, health related physical fitness and motor fitness components are important to everyone. However, more extensive development of these components may be required to achieve an appropriate level.

Norms is defined as Statistical tools which evaluate the status of an individual with respect to recently collected data on a large sample of a population group of the individual being examined. Most commonly used norms in physical education and human biology are the percentile ranks of a variable. Since, distance from average provides foundation for preparing standards of selection, there has been a general confusion between Norms and Standards among even many of the well qualified persons.

All these findings indicate that current physical education programs are inadequate to promote lifetime physical fitness. These findings have made physical educators realize that a change in curriculum is needed which would lead to development of attitude towards lifelong exercise behavior with emphasis on health related fitness.

Today, there is a growing emphasis on looking good, feeling good and living longer. Increasingly, scientific evidence tells us that one of the keys to achieving these ideals is fitness and exercise. Exercise is not just for Olympic hopefuls or supermodels. In fact, you're never too unfit, too young or too old to get started. Regardless of your age, gender or role in life, you can benefit from regular physical activity. If you're committed, exercise in combination with a sensible diet can help provide an overall sense of well- being and can even help prevent chronic illness, disability and premature death. One of the major rationales for promoting physical fitness in children is to development patterns of regular activity that can be maintained throughout life. Although the tracking coefficient for physical activity is not high, there is evidence that inactivity among children is linked to sedentary living among adults.. Involvement in physical activity as a number of physiological benefits for children, including positive changes in body composition, increased bone density, and improved ability to fight infection. Psychological benefits include a healthy development of self-concept, positive self- esteem, competence, and emotional wellbeing.

1.2 SCENARIO OF PHYSICAL EDUCATION IN INDIA VIS-À-VIS MAHARASHTRA

Physical Education developed on two different lines and through different channels. While sport, essentially a competitive phenomenon, achieved prominence due to an inevitably increasing impact of the Olympic Movement beginning in 1896, health and physical education (inclusive of sport in a limited way) were destined to become an ingredient of education first an extracurricular, then co- curricular and ultimately a curricular activity at school and college levels over time. Spread over one hundred years, the important landmarks in the development of physical education in India.

- *The **Mudaliar Commission** (1952-53) made a strong case for physical education by making the following recommendations:*

- *Physical education, group games and individual physical exercises should be given, no doubt, in the school under the supervision of Director of Physical Education........ We recommended that all teachers or at least those below the age of 40 should actively participate in many of the activities of physical education and thus make it a living part of the total school Programme instead of being a side issue entrusted to an isolated number of the staff......... We place special value on group games as they help to mould character of students in addition to affording recreational facilities and contributing to the physical well being.*

- *Realizing the importance of and having all praise for physical education, the **Kothari (Education) Commission,** in 1964-66 said :*

  ....it must be emphasized that such education contributes not only to physical fitness but also to physical efficiency, mental alertness, development of certain qualities like perseverance, team spirit, leadership, obedience, to rule, moderation in victory and balance in defeat............... physical education should include development exercises, rhythmic activity, sports and games, outing activities and group handling activities .... simpler activities should be introduced in eth early classes, more advanced ones should be gradually provided as boys and girls become more and more mature.

- *In its report, the **Ad-hoc Enquiry Committee on Games and Sports** (1958), headed by Late Maharaja Yadavindra Singh of Patiala, underscored the importance of physical education and insisted upon the physical education training institutions in the country to carry out a central plan of coaching. It recommended better sports facilities and funds for educational institutions,* *more attention to the nutritional status of the school children as a whole and special care for the talented boys and girls (Kamlesh , 2002)*

- *The Kaul-Kapoor committee, constituted by the All India Council of Sports, in 1961, inter alia stressed upon making physical education as an integral part of general education in schools and colleges. It required the educational institutions to thoroughly recognize their department of physical education. Emphasizing on the need to improve the sport infrastructure (play fields) in school and colleges, the Committee also recommended award of scholarships to outstanding young sports persons (Kamlesh, 2004)*

- *In several other documents, for example,* ***A National Plan of Physical Education,*** *1956 prepared by the Central Advisory Board of Physical Education and Recreation and approved by the Government of India, the "need for physical education in the educational institutions in the country" (Wakharkar,1991) was emphasized for its" very valuable contribution to our national life".*

1.3 RATIONAL OF THE STUDY

According to current thinking, Health Related Physical Fitness is concerned with the development of those qualities that offer protection against disease and frequently are associated with Physical activity. For example, certain physiological and psychological factors often affected by physical activity are thought to cause some degenerative disease. Thus health related physical fitness components are important to everyone. However, the degree of development health related physical fitness; a more extensive development of these components may be required to achieve an appropriate level. U.S Department of Health and Human Services: Promoting health / preventing Disease: Objectives for the nation, Washington, DC, 1980, U.S. Government Printing Office.

Keeping in view improving declined status of public health, world's leading institutions (American Academy of Physical Education, 1987, The American Academy of Pediatrics committee on Sports Medicine and School Health, 1987) and recent researchers (Berlin & Colditz, 1990, jopling 1988, Sallis & Mckenzie 1991, Smith, smith & Gilligan 1990, Simon-Morton et al.1987) have suggested that-

- Proper programme in physical education and its policy can cover 97% of the population for better public health.
- Appropriate physical activity in physical education can significantly reduce risk factors of stress related diseases.

This discussion presented above revealed that physical education has a social obligation of preparing the youth for work and socially useful activities. Literature also supports that children are naturally active and physical education provides an enjoyable way to educate them to sublimate their overall development.

Surprisingly, while going through the related literature and presently exited syllabi of schools prepared by Maharashtra State Board has been noted that though the health and fitness are the major objectives of physical Education, there is no proper procedure available for assessing the physical fitness of the school children.

It is revealed from the exiting syllabi of that Physical fitness teaching, training and evaluation has been incorporated and treated as an integral part of the present syllabus of Physical Education subject for school classes. However, there are no standard norms available for the assessment and Physical fitness till the date. Therefore the researcher has thought it appropriate to undertake this investigation which may help the concern professionals as well as authorities for its application and inclusion immediately. Further the problem to be investigated can also be justified by taking into consideration the fact that the Maharashtra Government has made the subject Physical Education at school level compulsory. However, the evaluation of the subject is being done by following the gradation system instead of inclusion of marks in being done by following the gradation system invested of inclusion of marks in their mark list. The researcher is quite sure that the findings of the present study would definitely enable him to recommend for the inclusion of marks in their marks list by providing objective and the reliable norms for the assessment of physical fitness of school children of Maharashtra. Hence there is an imminent need to undertake this research project.

1.4 RATIONALE OF PHYSICAL FITNESS AND HEALTH FOR CHILDREN

- **Concept of Physical Fitness**

Physical fitness is a general state of health and well-being and, more specifically, the ability to perform aspects of sports or occupations. Physical fitness is generally achieved through correct nutrition, exercise, hygiene and rest. It is a set of attributes or characteristics seen in people and which relate to the ability to perform a given set of physical activities.

Before the industrial revolution, fitness was the capacity to carry out the day's activities without undue fatigue. However with automation and changes in lifestyles physical fitness is now considered a measure of the body's ability to function efficiently and effectively in work and leisure activities, to be healthy, to resist hypokinetic diseases, and to meet emergency situations. (PCPFS Research Digests, 2014)

Individuals are physically fit when they can meet both the ordinary and the unusual demands of daily life safely and effectively without being overly fatigued and still have energy left for leisure and recreational activities. **Physical fitness** can be classified as health related, skill related, and physiological (Werner W. K. Hoeger, 2009).

- **Concept of Health Related Physical Fitness**

Health-related physical fitness is defined as fitness related to some aspect of health. This type of physical fitness is primarily influenced by an individual's exercise habits; thus, it is a dynamic state and may change. Physical characteristics that constitute health-related physical fitness include strength and endurance of skeletal muscles, joint flexibility, body composition, and cardio respiratory endurance. All these attributes change in response to appropriate physical conditioning programs, and all are related to health. (Werner W. K. Hoeger, 2009)

Health-related fitness is a physical state encompassing cardio respiratory endurance, muscular strength and endurance, muscular flexibility, and body composition are defined respectively as:

- ***Cardio respiratory endurance:*** the ability of the heart, lungs, and blood vessels to supply oxygen to the cells to meet the demands of prolonged physical activity (also referred to as aerobic exercise)
- ***Muscular strength and endurance:*** the ability of the muscles to generate force
- ***Muscular strength:*** Ability to exert maximum force against resistance.
- ***Muscular endurance:*** Ability of a muscle to exert sub-maximal force repeatedly over a period of time.
- ***Muscular flexibility:*** the achievable range of motion at a joint
- ***Body composition:*** the amount of lean body mass and adipose tissue (fat mass) in the human body

Many studies have strongly supported the hypothesis that sedentary habits increase the risk of premature death, primarily due to higher rates of cardiovascular disease.

An approach to studying the impact of inactivity on health would be to examine the relation of physical fitness to disease and death rates. The primary determinant of physical fitness is physical activity, although heredity also makes a contribution. In fact, physical fitness can be used as a marker for physical activity level. The major advantage of using physical fitness in risk assessment is that it can be measured objectively.

1.5 HEALTH - EFFECTS OF ACTIVITY AND FITNESS IN CHILDREN

The major apparent health benefit of a fit and active way of life is reduced risk of developing several chronic diseases.

First, some medical problems, such as insulin -dependent diabetes and obesity and its attendant complications can be alleviated by appropriate exercise. Second physical activity may benefit young people is to help maintain proper growth. It is believed that a certain amount of exercise is necessary for growth, although the specifics are not known. Finally, the most important contribution children's physical activity can make is to influence their lifetime exercise pattern positively. Exercise and health interrelationships across the lifespan are illustrated in Figure.

If childhood exercise, however, can increase the likelihood that a person will maintain physical activity into and through adulthood, significant health benefits are possible.

Exercise- Health Relationship

The natural state of human beings is to be physically active. Objective measures of physical fitness confirm that children are, on average, the most physically fit group in our society. Unfortunately as the regions of inactive adults prove, we are successful in engineering activity out of modern life and we train children to be sedentary.

Many studies strongly support the hypothesis that sedentary habits increase the risk of premature death, primarily due to so higher rates of cardiovascular diseases (Blair & Meredith, 1994).

Physical activity influences can be categorized as biological, psychological, social, and environmental. All of these factors are associated with children's physical activity, so effective interventions must operate on multiple levels. No single approach is likely to be effective, and children's needs change with age. Special attention should be devoted to girls and to adolescents, because their activity levels are relatively low, and to economically disadvantaged youth, because they have access to fewer facilities and programs. Based on the results of the determinants research, 15 recommendations (Pate & Russell) were made for physical educators who hope to be successful in promoting physical activity in their students.

Physical education can be defined as more than "letting the kids blow off stream" or teaching basic skills Physical education should prepare children for a lifetime physical activity, just as other teachers prepare children for a lifetime of learning and work. Children should not become dependant on PE for their physical activity.

Influences on Children's physical activity

There are several health benefits of regular physical activity. An important issue in promoting physical activity concerns understanding the determinants and changing behaviour. This has two key factors,

- **Personal factors**

  Biological and psychological characteristics

- **Environmental factors**

  Social and physical environment

Determinants of Physical Activity in Children and Adolescents

Determinants are variables that are correlated with physical activity and they may have casual effects. The most promising models hypothesize that behavior is influenced by intrapersonal, social and physical environmental variables. Some determinants, such as age, sex, race and ethnicity, and genetics are not modifiable but can identify groups at risk for being inactive. It may be more important to identify modifiable determinants that can be used to guide the design of all sub groups. Important modifiable determinants for young people include self-efficacy, enjoyment, social support from family and friends, and for young children, time spent outdoors, Physical Education, sports teams and activity classes can provide substantial amount of physical activity for young people.

1.6 STATEMENT OF THE PROBLEM

Consulting related literature on the present status of physical education in schools in India and on the basis of long standing professional experiences in the field of physical education, the present researcher is in opinion that there is no information available till- to-date about the standard norms of health-related physical fitness of school children in India. It will be, therefore, considered appropriate by the investigator to develop the standard norms of health-related physical fitness for school children. The problems stated above indicate that there is an imminent need to conduct research in the area of school health programme. Therefore, the present study entitled, "***Establishment of Norms for Health Related Physical Fitness for School Children***

aged 13-15 of Maharashtra State" has been undertaken.

1.7 SIGNIFICANCE OF THE STUDY

This research project is significance because –

- Norms of the 'Health Related Physical Fitness' may help to categorize /classify the students in forming a homogeneous group judiciously for competition.
- Physical education teacher and sports coaches may get a standardization test for measuring the fitness status of their students and develop the relationship with health status as well.
- The students having good level of 'Health Related Physical fitness' may be directed for specified sports training to enrich top performance.
- This study, may be helping the present status of Health Related Physical Fitness of students.
- At present there is no norms therefore it may be helpful to construct the norms.
- It may be helpful and imp limitation of physical education program.

1.8 OBJECTIVES OF THE STUDY

The research study has been conducted with the following objectives:

- To design some 'test-items' for measuring Health Related Physical Fitness Test.
- To standardize a "Health Related Physical Fitness Test" for the students of secondary school level students;
- To establish the norms of the Health Related Physical Fitness for the secondary school children of Maharashtra state;
- To establish and standardize an accurate 'system of evaluation' of physical education suitable, specifically for the students of age group 13 to 15 years of Maharashtra state.
- To determine the norms of the 'system of evaluation' in relation to the competencies or outcomes of physical education of the students of age group 13 to 15 years of Maharashtra state.
- To validate the norms in the process of the evaluation.

1.9 HYPOTHESIS OF THE STUDY

On the basis of the available literature, it has been hypothesized that-

H01: The *'Health Related Physical Fitness Test'* is not having sufficient degree of reliability and validity especially for the student's age group 13 to 15 years of Maharashtra state.

H02: The *'Health Related Physical Fitness Test'* is not having significant level of normality in data especially for the student's age group 13 to 15 years of Maharashtra state.

1.10 LIMITATIONS OF THE STUDY

While conducting this study, the researcher recorded the following shortcomings:

- As the subjects selected for the study, were randomly selected from various Schools situated in 8 educational zones in Maharashtra, the factors viz., geographical conditions, diet, nutrition, and such other factors that might affect this normative study, could not be controlled by the present researcher.
- The investigator could not attend all the schools situated in education zones.

1.11 DELIMITATION OF THE STUDY

This study has a very wide scope, because it has been designed in such a way so that it will help other researcher, scholars, sports scientists and physical education teachers to conduct similar studies. However, this study has been delimited considering the followings:

1. The present study has been delimited to the both boys and girls studying in the schools of Maharashtra.
2. The present study has been selected test of Health Related Physical Fitness component.
3. The students studying in Standards VII, VIII and IX in the state of Maharashtra.
4. Selected districts from the educational zones of Maharashtra.

1.12 DEFINITIONS OF THE TERMS AND CONCEPTS

- **Health**

It is a state of complete physical, mental, social, spiritual well-being and not merely the absence of disease.

- **Fitness**

Its condition that helps us look, feel and do our best without undue fatigue.

- **Exercise**

It is a physical activity of exerting one's muscles in various ways to keep fit.

- **Norms**

The status quo of defined group in the form in statistical constants in other words norms provide scoring scale, say in the percentiles of a defined population group.

- **Health Related Physical Fitness**

Capacity of an individual to perform specific physical task involving muscular effects. Physical fitness various considerably in different people and in the same person from time to time.

- **Test**

A test is a form of questioning and / or measuring used to assess retention of knowledge and capability or to measure able in some physical endeavor. It is a specific tool, Procedure or technique used to elicit a response from the students in order to gain information to be used as a basis for appraisal of the quality or quantity of elements such as, fitness, skill, knowledge, values etc.

- **Measurement**

Measurement is a technique of evaluation, with uses tests and other procedures and instruments precisely with objectivity. It gives quantitative data and characteristically can express its results in numerical from that indicating ability of capacity involving fitness, motor skill, knowledge, value or process etc.

- **Muscular strength**

The maximal force that a muscle or a muscle group can generate in a single effort.

- **Muscular Endurance**

Ability of a muscles group of contract over an extended time against moderate resistance.

- **Cardiovascular Endurance**

It may be defined as the ability of heart and lungs to take in and to transport adequate amounts of oxygen to the working muscle for activities that involve large muscle masses, to be performed over a long period of time e.g., running, swimming etc.

- **Flexibility**

Flexibility is the ability to perform movement with greater range of the motion of large amplitude.

- **Body composition**

The relative properties of fat-free (lean) tissue in the body. Commonly reported as "percent body fat," thus identifying the proposition of the total body mass is then determined as the balance of the total body mass.

CHAPTER
II

CHAPTER-II

REVIEW OF RELATED LITERATURE

2.1 INTRODUCTION

Review of the related literature gives valuable insight to the investigator regarding the problem that to be solved. The collected studies have been presented in a chronological order here as under:

2.2 STUDIES ON DEVELOPMENT OF TESTS AND CONSTRUCTION OF NORMS

R. K. Sharma, (2014) conducted a study on constructing of Norms for selected Physical Fitness Test Battery as a Gauge for Sports Potential among Kabaddi Players. The purpose of this study was to construct norms for selected physical fitness test battery as a gauge for sports potential among kabaddi players. For the purpose of the present study, sixty (N=60), male kabaddi players of Punjabi University, Patiala between the age group of 18-25 years volunteered to participate in the study. The Handgrip Strength Test was used to measure Muscular Strength, Vertical Jump Test was used to measure Muscular Power, Chin up Test was used to measure Muscular Endurance, 20 Meter Dash Test was used to measure Running Speed, Illinois Agility Test was used to measure Running Agility, Standing Long Jump Test was used to measure Jumping Ability, Overhead Medicine Ball Throw test was used to measure Throwing Ability, Sit and Reach Flexibility Test was used to measure Flexibility and Stork Balance Stand Test was used to measure Balance. In order to construct the norms, Percentile Scale was used. Further, the scores were classified into five grades i.e., very good, good, average, poor and very poor.

Kosa, (2014) constructed a Health-Related Physical Fitness Norms for Students of Rajamangala University of Technology Thanyaburi. The purpose of this research was to construct health-related physical fitness norms for students of Rajamangala University of Technology Thanyaburi. The sample used in this research was 410 male and 460 female students who were studying in the first semester of academic year 2006 at Rajamangala University of Technology Thanyaburi. The instrument was the AAHPERD Health-Related Physical Fitness Test which consisted of three items: sit and reach, one minute sit-up, 1.5 mile run/walk, and the ACSM Fitness Test consisting of body mass index. The data were analyzed by mean, standard deviation, percentage and norms using raw scores. The norms were divided into five levels: excellent, good, moderate, low and poor. It was found that the health-related physical fitness norms for male and female students of Rajamangala University of Technology Thanyaburi by using physical fitness tests: body mass index, sit and reach, one minute sit-up and 1.5 mile run/walk were at moderate level. The research provided health-related physical fitness norms for students of Rajamangala University of Technology, Thanyaburi.

Jagathesan, (2013) purposed a study was to construct the norms for evaluating performance of players in the game of Kabaddi. For this purpose, four hundred male college level Kabaddi players were randomly selected from various colleges of Tamilnadu state, India and their age ranged from 18 to 20 years. The performance of Kabaddi players was assessed by Skill Test Battery constructed by Jagathesan and Ganeshkumar was chosen for this study. The data, which was collected by administering tests, was statistically treated to develop norms for all the test items. The norms were constructed by using percentile and 6 sigma scale techniques analyzed through SPSS. The results of the study revealed that the scores were further classified into five grades i.e. excellent, good, average, satisfactory and poor.

Uppal, (2012) constructed a physical fitness Test for High School Boys : A Factor Analytic Approach. The study intends to develop physical fitness test battery for high school boys. The physical fitness standards and norms diverge from place to place, region to region, geographical locations, food habits etc. The physical fitness standards set for one country may not be suitable for another country. The study was taken keeping in view of Indian scholastic conditions. Thirty two physical fitness test items were preferred or tailored by considering the appearance authority of test items and experts' judgment in the field of physical education. These variables were administered to 180 high school sports boys who had represented their relevant schools at least in Inter School, Taluk Level sport competitions. The data was subjected to principal component factor analysis by using SPSS software. Factor analytic results acquiesced seven factors, which accounted for 69.3 percent of the entire variance in the data set. Six components of physical fitness were identified of which the muscular strength emerged as principal component (with 34.0 percent of total variance) physical fitness. A test battery of six items was developed by considering rotated factor loadings, reliability and objectivity of test variables. The constructed test measures muscular strength, muscular endurance, agility, explosive power and speed of limb factors of high school boys.

Saha, (2018) compared the Health Related Physical Fitness variables and psychomotor ability between rural and urban school going children. One thousand students age ranging from 17 to 30 years were selected as subjects for the study of which five hundred were Tribal and the remaining five hundred were Non-tribal School going from different schools of North 24 Parganas District, West Bengal. The subjects were tested in their respective school ground for continuously five days. The criterion measures included under Health related physical fitness directly related to improvement of health are 1) Sit and Reach test to measure lower back flexibility and was, 2) Body Fat Monitor, an electronic device manufactured by Omron model no. HBF 306 to measure Body fat percentage, 3) Aerobic /cardiovascular function was measured by the 1.5 mile run test, 4) Abdominal muscular strength and endurance was used measured by Partial Curl Ups and 5) Upper body muscular strength and endurance was measured by Right Angle Push- Ups. To measure the Psychomotor ability, reaction ability was considered and wasmeasured by Nelson Hand Reaction Test. For the purpose of Comparison of Health related physical fitness variables and Psychomotor ability between Rural and Urban School going children, Student's 't' ratio statistical technique was used (SPSS Version 18) to analyse the data. The level of significance was set at $p<0.05$ level. The results showed significant differences between Rural and Urban school going children in all the Health related Physical fitness components as well as in Reaction ability under psychomotor ability and rural school going children was found better than urban school going children.

Abidalhussain, Bin, Lian, & Ali, (2012) compared the study on relations between health- related physical fitness, physical activity, and BMI among children in Selangor, Malaysia. This study aim was to investigate the relation between health-related physical fitness (HRF), physical activity (PA), and BMI among children in Malaysia. PA was measured and classified into three levels based on the checklist questions. Anthropometric and HRF were measured in a sample of 918 students. BMI was computed and classified into underweight, normal, overweight/obese. The results of the study shows that, more boys than girls were underweight and overweight (14.8% vs 12.4%), (28.8% vs 19.4%). Boys perform significantly ($P< 0.000$) better than girls in all HRF except for the sit-and-reach. All HRF tests were significantly correlated with each other in boys and girls, but BMI was weakly correlated with sit-and-reach in boys, and sit-and-reach and sit-up girls. Boys and girls performances decrease (p for trend < 0.05) in all HRF tests from normal weight to overweight/obese. Overweight/underweight children had poorer performance in HRF than normal weight children. However, performances of overweight and underweight children in high PA level were significantly better in overall HRF tests than their low PA level.

Monyeki, (2012) studied on health-related fitness, body composition and physical activity status among adolescent learners: The PAHL study. Physical inactivity (PI) is found to be a major contributor to the high incidence of overweight and obesity among children and adolescents. As such, PI was significantly related to risk factors of cardiovascular disease. Studies especially in the 14-years in adolescents' learners are sparse. The purpose of this study was to determine the health-related physical fitness (HRPF), body composition and physical activity (PA) status among adolescent learners. A total of 283 adolescents learners (111 boys and 172 girls) with mean age of 14.90±0.72 years from the Physical Activity and Health Longitudinal Study (PAHLS) were participants in the study. Body composition according to the standard procedures of the International Society for the Advancement of Kinanthropometry (ISAK), HRPF using the Eurofit protocol test and PA levels using the International Physical Activity Questionnaire (IPAQ) were assessed and administered. Subsequently, total PA scores were calculated. The results show that on average, the boys (165.41±9.55cm) were significantly taller than the girls (157.88±6.94cm) ($p<0.000$). Girls had a slightly higher significant BMI (21.43±4.37 kg/m^2) than the boys (20.01±3.71kg/m^2) ($p=0.002$). When the learners were categorised based on their BMI scores, the girls were more overweight (32.4%) compared to the boys (17.1%). Additionally, the girls (%body fat 26.01±8.51) were substantially ($p<0.000$) fatter than the boys (13.19±8.56). Furthermore, the results also indicated that the boys had consistently better performances in all the HRPF tests than the girls (p<0.000). More girls (19%) than boys (16%) watched TV for more than 3 hours daily. A total of 85 (30%), 78(27.5%) and 88(31.1%) of the adolescent students had low, moderate and high PA involvement.

Verma, (2011) purposed the study was to develop the physical profile of Kabaddi players. A sample consists of 100 male Kabaddi players. They were selected from West-Zone Inter-University championship as the subjects of the study. Their age ranged between 18 to 23 years. Keeping the feasibility in mind, speed, agility and explosive was selected for this study. Speed and agility were assessed by administering 50 yard dash and the performance was recorded in seconds and shuttle run respectively. To determine for the explosive power, standing board jump was used and the reading was recorded in meters. To develop the physical profile of Kabaddi players, descriptive analysis was applied. The results of the study indicates that in case of 50 yard dash, standing broad jump and shuttle run Kabaddi Players were having average in scores. In case of standing broad jump Kabaddi Players scored above average. It was found that West-Zone University Kabaddi players were average in speed and shuttle run and in case of standing broad jump were above the average.

Mohite, (2011) studied on computing Physical Fitness Norms for Girls of Junior Colleges in Barshi Taluka. The purpose of the study was to determine the physical fitness ability and to comport the norms of selected physical fitness components for the women students of junior colleges. The subjects were classified according to their physical ability in the selected physical fitness components of women students for the purpose of the teaching and coaching. The norms of the physical fitness of women student of the junior college of Barshi Taluka was bear sufficient reliability. The source of data and the procedure adopted for the selection and the administration of the physical fitness test and statistical technique for construction the physical fitness norms. Used AAHPER Youth fitness test used and the following items for girls 1. Push Up 2. Bend knee sit-up 3. Standing broad jump 4. 50 Mtr. Running 5. 40 Mtr. Shuttle run 6. 600 Mtr.run & walk. The new set of norms was constructed by using the T Scale method and the score were given in the T Scale norms. The result of the study was prepared suitable norms to evaluate the student's performance through a selected physical fitness test. The norms in physical fitness for girls the junior college in Barshi Taluka were prepared which could be used for grading students in this aspects of required program of physical education in curriculum.

Purashwani & Purashwani, (2010) studied to construct the norms for evaluating performance of players in Table Tennis Skill Test. Since, there was a lack of standardized evaluative criteria in Table Tennis for assessing the ability, grading and predicting the performance of Table-Tennis players, an effort was undertaken to construct Norms for Skill Test for junior and senior Table Tennis Players. For this purpose 816 male, 410 Junior and 406 Senior, state and national level Table-Tennis players of different states in India were randomly selected to serve as subjects. The performance of Table Tennis players in Table Tennis test battery of four test items, namely, Alternate Push Test, Target Service Test, Alternate Counter Test and Fore Hand Drive on Target Test with foot movement after playing backhand push, constructed by Pushpendra Purashwani and Dr. A.K. Datta, were chosen for the purpose of the study. The data was collected by administering the test for the selected test items during the Summer Coaching Camps and Regular Training Sessions of various districts, different Ranking Table Tennis Tournaments and State and Inter-District Table-Tennis Championships in the year 2006. The data, which was collected by administering tests, was statistically treated to develop norms for all the test items. The two normative scales, namely, the Percentile Scale and 7 Sigma Scale were constructed for the junior and senior table tennis players of state and national level. The norms were constructed by using Percentile and 7 Sigma Scale techniques analyzed through statistical packages, the scores were further classified into five grades i.e. very good, good, average, poor and very poor under Normal Distribution.

Guleria, (2027) developed athletic norms for senior secondary school boys and girls students of Himachal Pradesh. A sample of 2400 subjects, 1200 boys and 1200 girls, with the age of 17+ to 18+ was selected from forty eight senior secondary schools. Only selected athletic events as per Himachal Pradesh school education board's syllabus for XI and XII was considered for the study. Performances of subjects in athletic events were used for construction of norms. Obtained scores from subjects were converted in Z score, T score, percentile and sigma scale for construction of norms.

Singh, (2006) conducted a study on construction and standardization of specific skill test battery for male handball players. A sample of 600 male School, University and Senior levels handball players, 200 in each category were selected for the study. The study had two phases. In first phase selected 15 test items were sent to 30 experts of consideration also reliability was established. In the second Phase, data were collected through nine test items, Catching (Score), Passing (Score), Passing (Time), Throwing (Score), Throwing (Time), Shooting (Score), Shooting (Time), Footwork (Score), Dribbling (Time) and norms were constructed with the help of established test on 594 male Handball Players. The Percentile scale was applied for construction of norms.

Dutt, (2005) investigated on health related physical fitness of boys aged 8 to 18 years. The investigation was carried out on 797 male children and youth belonging to Punjab and falling in the age range of 8 to 18 years. Four components of health related physical fitness namely cardiovascular endurance, muscular strength/endurance, flexibility and body composition were assessed using standard techniques. The results in general indicate a trend of improvement in cardio respiratory fitness of the boys belonging to the study with increase in age. However when comparison was made with Prudential fitness gram standards Results indicate poor level of Vo2 max in boys of the present study, the results of muscular strength and endurance, an important health related component of fitness indicate variations in its development with respect to different body regions in boys of the present study from age 8 to 18 years. The muscles related to the upper body region like triceps, deltoid, pectorals major etc. are observed to develop relatively better in their strength endurance ability than the muscles belonging to abdominal, hip and leg regions. It was believed that disproportionate development of muscular strength endurance in boys of the study may be due to their habitual life style and a craze for some selected muscular strengthening exercises, like use of dumbbells, lifting weights etc. in order to develop their body for an attractive physical appearance. Average percent body fat of these boys at all age level was observed to fall in the health fitness zone. However the percent body fat of boys of the study after the age of 14 years and onwards exhibit a sharp rise, which continues up to 17 years of age.

Marshall, Smith, & Bauman, (2005) examined a reliability and validity of a brief physical activity assessment tool suitable for doctors and it was used to identify inactive patients in the primary care setting. The researcher examined volunteer eight family doctors, screened consenting patients for physical activity participation using a brief physical activity assessment tool. Inter rater reliability was assessed within one week on seventy one. Validity was assessed against an objective physical activity monitor computer science and applications accelerometer with forty two subjects. Researcher was found the brief physical activity assessment tool was reliable instrument, with validity similar to that of more detailed self report measures of physical activity. It was a tool that can be used efficiently in routine primary health care services to identify insufficiently active patients who may need physical activity advice.

Lemmink & Elferink, (2004) evaluated a study of reliability of the field hockey specific sprints and dribble tests among field hockey players. Determined the reliability of two field Hockey specific tests were: (1) The Shuttle Sprint and Dribble Test (2) Slalom sprint and Dribble Test. Data were collected from twenty two young male and twelve female Hockey players. The data was assessed on two occasions within four weeks period and concluded that both the tests are reliable measures of sprint and dribble performance of young field Hockey players.

Kaur, (2003) evaluated a study of motor abilities test are reliable and valid for testing the subject. Seventy secondary school female volleyball players were selected as subjects. Each subject was administered with eleven motor abilities tests

i.e. Standing Broad Jump, Medicine Ball Throw, 50m Sprint, Forward Bend Reach, Sit-ups, 10 x 4 Metre Shuttle Run, 800 Meter Run, Right Hand Grip Strength, Left Hand Grip Strength, Vertical Jump and Pushups. For assessing playing abilities five test were administered i.e. Upper Hand Pass, Under Hand Pass, Target Pass, Service and Wall 25 Volley Tests. A composite score of motor ability and playing ability was made differently and each test was co-related with it to find out the validity. For reliability, test re-test score was correlated with each other. It was found that all tests were quite reliable and valid.

Yadav, (2002) developed a specific physical fitness test and constructed norms for National level male judokas with a sample of 200 judokas who represent different states and paramilitary forces of northern India. The study had two phases. In first phase selected 22 test items were administered on 160 judokas of national level players before their major competition. The test battery consisted of six items, namely Right hand grip strength, Sit and reach, Sit ups, 30 Meter run, Standing Broad Jump and Pull–ups with scientific authenticity. In the second phase, norms were constructed with the help of established test on 200 male judokas. The T-scale, hull scale and sigma scale were applied for construction of norms.

Dinesh, (1998) conducted a study to evolve physical fitness norms on various items of Fleishman's fitness battery for high and higher secondary school boys of Himachal Pradesh and also to evaluate the physical fitness level of the secondary school male students of Himachal Pradesh. To accomplish the study 3,840 students between the age group of 13 to 16 years were randomly selected from both the urban and rural area. The results of the study shows that there was a significant difference from fifteen years to sixteen years male subjects of Himachal Pradesh in almost all fitness components. The boys of 16 years age were found significantly superior than 15 years to 13 year boys. The fifteen boys were better than 14 and 13 years boys. Similarly 14 years boys were superior then 13 year boys in all the components of Fleishman's test battery. The result of the study has also shown that the male subjects of rural areas were significantly superior than urban subjects in six of ten fitness components of Fleishman's test battery.

Anayanwa, (1997) attempted to establish physical fitness norms for Nigerian boys and girls in the age group 11 years to 18 years. The study included the following test items shuttle run, push-ups for boys, chair push-ups for girls : flexed knee sit ups: 45 meter dash; standing long jump; pull-ups for boys; flexed arms hang for girls; a minute run for subjects 13 to 18 years: The results of the study shows that high correlations were obtained on the test re-test method. The test items were considered objectives. The activities can be accepted as true test items for the component of physical fitness, which they support to measure. In most of the test items the performance of the boys improved from the lower to upper age level. The boys performed better than girls in all the test activities. (5) The mean score revalued that the girls of lower age level tend to posses better physical fitness status than the girls of the upper levels.

Bitcon, (1995) had constructed a norm table for the grades of 9–12 by taking the following test. Pull–ups, two minutes sit ups, standing broad jump and 300 meters run. Researcher showed the comparison of the validity of the test against with AAPHER youth fitness test. The obtained validity and the reliability co– efficient were 0.934 and 0.961 respectively.

Desouza, (1993) conducted a research on standardization on norms for physical fitness tests for girls in the age group of 13 to 16 years in the state of Goa. The purpose of this study was to standardize norms for physical fitness tests for in the age group of 13 to 16 years in the state of Goa, and also to compare the physical fitness status of the girls in the different age groups. The physical fitness components considered for this study were strength (vertical and standing broad jump), muscular endurance (flexed arm hang), C.V. endurance (50m dash), agility (4x10m shuttle run), and flexibility (bend, touch and twist). The researcher propose to administer the test to about 4000 girls in the age groups of 13, 14, 15 and 16 years taking about 1000 girls in each age group from about 75 schools of all the 11 Talukas in Goa. Seven test items in the test battery were split up into two sets and were conducted on two consecutive days. The data collected on the subjects in respect of different physical fitness items was utilized for constructing the Percentile scale, Sigma scale and Hull scale-test employed for comparing subjects representing different age groups in various test items considered in the study. The level of significance was set at 0.05 level of confidence. There was no significant difference in the physical fitness of the girls (13 to 16 yr.) from the state of Goa. The subjects belonging to the 15 years age group were found to be significantly superior to that of 13 years age group in vertical jumping ability. Dorothy (1961) 40 evolved norms of physical fitness for college women from 57 college and the data of 3300 subjects were collected for seven test items. In order to be consistent with the percentile norms were calculated from 0 to 100 at an interval of 5.

Jackson & Jeffrey, (1992) intended to investigate the reliability and validity of one mile walk as field test for aerobic capacity and to develop norms for the test. For establishing reliability and validity the samples included 41 males (n = 21) and females (n = 20) with the age group of 19 – 32 years. The subjects performed the treadmill stress tests to determine the peak O2 consumption and 3 trails of maximum one mile walk on an indoor track. The mean trail reliability estimate was 0.96 but a significant trend was present. The correlation 'r' value between trail 3rd and peak O2 consumption was 0.57. When the rock port prediction function using age, weight, gender, one mile walk and ending heart rate was used to predict peak O2 the improved to 0.66. The normative samples included males (n=400) and females (n=426) with an age range of 18–30 years. They performed a practice trail of one mile walk followed by a performance trail. The percentile norm was constructed. The AAHPERD health related fitness norms published in 1980 were based on over 12,000 boys and girls. A cluster sample representing several geographic regions was followed in 1985 and the results of National children and youth fitness study was published in the January 1985 issue of the journal of Physical Education Recreation and dance over 8,500 boys and girls in grades 5 to 12 were administered health related and motor fitness tests. This represented a national probability sample with few exceptions for selected age groups. The children that comprised the 1980 health related physical fitness test sample were more fit than 1985 Naeyes sample.

Pillai, (1991) studied on computation of norms for 12-minute run and walk among school boys. In this study, the researcher described cardio-vascular endurance as one of the basic and important components of physical fitness, A state level norm would be useful for boys to understand their present status compared with other boys of the same age, for the teacher and coach either to understand or to prescribe a programme to improve the student ability and to compare it with other states. Since 15,000 subjects were involved in the study, 12-minutes walk test was considered as the more appropriate test for assessing cardiovascular endurance. For this study, data was collected from 20 districts except the Nilgris district. Data collected from 250 subjects in each age category of 13, 14 and 15 years school boys. Tests were conducted on 12-minutes run/walk and the distance covered the nearest 50th meter were recorded as their performance. Two-way analysis of variance was applied to find out whether there was any significant difference between the district and age group in 12-minutes run/walk performance. It was found that significant difference was noticed only among different age groups. Hence, norms were constructed throughout the state for different age groups by using Hull scale. Height, weight and twenty eight tests commonly used to measure strength were administered by Avent (1964) 24 to 101 nine and ten years old and 100 eleven and twelve year old Caucasian girls. Regression equations were set up for estimating the following: general static strength based on McCloy's unweighted strength score and dynomertrical measures: general dynamic strength based on the average of T-scores of five dynamic strength measures and ten dynamic strength variables; and total static and dynamic strength based on the overage of T-scores derived from dynamometrical measures and the five-item dynamic strength measures. Norms were established.

Kaur D, (1989) developed a study on physical fitness norms for the high school girls of Punjab state belonging to the age group of 12 to 15 years. The samples were selected from the various urban and rural school of Punjab State. Sample consisted of four thousand students by using Fleishman's Test Battery. In this study, the researcher conducted the lower performance level of rural students in most of the physical fitness variables as compared to their urban counter parts. The percentile norms for physical fitness test were valid and suitable to assess the physical fitness level of school girls. Researcher observed that the subjects belonging to urban residence were significantly superior to rural subject in terms of dynamic flexibility, arm and shoulder strength and trunk strength variables. But, the results were not found to be significant between the urban and rural girls again extent flexibility, speed of change of direction, endurance level of arms and shoulders, co-ordinate agility, cardiovascular endurance and speed of running. The four age steps were found significantly different from each other against most of the physical fitness variables, while there were no significant differences in a few variables between some age steps.

Singh P., (1988) had taken a normative study of the Physical Fitness of Male Teenagers of the State of Jammu and Kashmir in the ages 13 through 19 years. The variables considered were, pull-ups (arm and shoulder girdle strength) bent knee sit-ups (abdominal strength) standing broad jump (explosive strength) 50 meters dash (speed) shuttle run (agility) and 600 meters run walk (cardio-vascular endurance). The researcher concluded that the subjects belonging to age group 16 through 19 years showed better performances in all variables over the other age group of 13 through 15 years.

Yadav B., (1986) conducted a study on standardization of physical fitness norms for the school children of Haryana (13 to 16 Years of age) with the purpose of estimating the fitness and comparing the standard of physical fitness of urban and rural boys of Haryana. For the purpose of this study 3600 school boys of the twelve districts of Haryana state were randomly selected and the performance of the boys were recorded on 50mts dash, shotput, standing broad jump, zig zag run, situps and step up tests. The norms in terms of percentile rank of said group were developed.

Singh R. M., (1986) developed physical fitness norms of Punjab State high school boys. Researcher randomly selected five thousand school boys of Punjab state. The sample included rural and urban subjects in equal number for the collection of in data. The researcher included test items such as standing broad jump, sit and reach test, agility run, sit-up bent knee, 50 meter dash, push-ups(chair), cricket ball throw, 600-meter run walk. The researcher observed significant difference in number of test items between urban and rural school boys. Significant difference relationship between age and performance of the subjects was also observed. The test items were standardized through the development of percentile norms which was found to be suitable to access the physical fitness of Punjab state high school boys ranging between 12 to 15 years of age.

Singh A., (1986) conducted a normative study of physical fitness of Punjab university men students. The researcher applied Fleishman's Test Battery or four thousand male students belonging to the various colleges affiliated to Punjab University to collect the data. The students ranged between 17 to 22 years of age. The researcher found linearity of physical fitness status according to age. The students of rural areas were significantly superior in all the test items than urban students. The researcher developed percentile norms and established their reliability, subjective and validity.

Blair & Pate, (1983) conducted a study on health-related physical fitness test. Testing 12,000 children from age five to seventeen in Seventeen States developed percentile norms. Volunteer physical education teachers administered tests excepting the skinfolds in standardized manner. Percentile norms for the skinfold test were obtained from the national health examination survey.

Barbante, (l983) conducted a study on Brazilian boys and girls. The purpose of this investigation was to determine the status of physical fitness of selected Brazilian boys and girls and to provide norms for Brazilian school children from the scores achieved on selected physical fitness tests and to find out difference between performance of Brazilian boys and girls and to determine if difference existed between norms for Brazilian and American boys and girls for selected physical fitness measurements. 342 boys and girls were taken as samples who were enrolled in a public school system in Brazil during 1982 year. Results of the study shows that selected Brazilian Schools Populations age group from 6 to 14 years, height and weight of both sexes increased at approximately at the same rate. Girls were significantly taller and heavier than boys during adolescence. 2. Brazilian girls had higher values than boys for triceps and sub-scapular skin fold measurements, sit- ups and in reach test. 3. Brazilian boys performed better than Brazilian girl in modified sit-ups tests, nine minute run test, 12 minute test, 50 meter dash test and standing long jump test 4) The comparison between norms for Brazilian and American boys and girls showed that American boys and girls in general were taller and heavier and had a higher scores in standing long jump.

Sittmann, (1981) prepared norms for North-East Missouri State University students of health and physical fitness concept classes. In which 372 male and 648 female subjects were tested. The test conducted was the sum of 6 skin folds, predicted percent fat, predicted VO2 max, grip strength; leg strength, back strength, vertical jump distance and vertical jump power. Statistic used was mean, standard deviations and range of all variables. Classification was based on sex. Percentiles in increments of 5 were constructed for each variable in each classification.

Jackson H. A, (1980) conducted a study on physical fitness. The norms-reflected standards were developed from scores of over 1500 men and women, who were tested at different Young Men's Christian Association throughout the United States. The standards included the test scores associated with selected percentiles. A percentile was the percentage of people of a given age group and gender who achieved the score. A maximal oxygen uptake of 54ml/kg. Minimum fell in the ninety fifth percentiles for men in the age group of thirty five years and below. This means that of all men tested who have 35 years and younger ninety five per cent had an average score of 54ml/kg. Minimum or lower and only five per cent had an average score of more than 54ml/kg. Minimum.

Das, (1980) constructed norms in Physical Fitness Tests for boys of class 9-11 of Government School of Delhi with the purpose of computing a norm for evaluating performance in physical fitness as required in the curriculum for the required programme of physical education. AAHPERD Youth Fitness Test and N.P.F.D. Battery 'A' were administered and norms were worked out. A comparison of obtained data with American student's shows that Indian students seem to be poor in abdominal strength and shoulder girdles strength.

Falls, (1979) established norms on the AAHPERD youth physical fitness. The norms were computed for more than 10,000 young subjects. Those who fall below the 50th percentile in any area were advised to participate in a fitness- developed programme Physical Performance test was selected by Fleishman 27 in 1964 on the basic of the factors isolated from much larger batteries of tests. Fleishman reviewed the previously published literature in the field of physical fitness and added by his own personal experience in presetting and pilot, studies. The researcher selected a battery of 30 test items generally considered to be measure of strength and another battery of 30 test items hypothesized to be measure of speed, flexibility, balance and co-ordination. Norms, or standards performance scores, were developed for boys and girls between the age of 15 to 18 years on the basic of the score scores for more than 2,000 students for most of the tests.

Watson, (1978) established norms for Nebraska boys and girls. The tests selected for Neb Eel physical fitness test were standing long jump or vertical jump, 50 yard dash, sit-ups, stick jump and 300 yards distance run. The tests for secondary test were pull-ups or flexed arm hang, 50 yard dash, standing long jump, sit-ups, side step and mile or 9 minute run or 12 minute run. The sample was selected randomly. One-percent sample was selected from Neb schools to establishment of norms. The norms were established for each test for girls, boys and groups according to chronological age. Percentile statistic was used.

Robson, (1978) had conducted a study on a simple physical fitness test battery for elementary school children. They took 152 boys and 150 girls of Kendriya

Vidyalaya, Gwalior. The test battery was practicable and simpler than the existing physical fitness test and measures most of the essential motor qualities of elementary school children. The norms were prepared for the selected items and can be used for classifying the children into ability groups by assessing their physical fitness.

Zuti, (1977) prepared physical fitness norms for college freshmen. The age group selected for this was from 17.6, 18.5 to 19.5 years from freshmen of Kansas State University. The total subjects were 3000. The test was conducted for strength test, flexibility body composition, and cardio-vascular fitness. The result shows that the college freshmen at Kansas State University were above average and standards were appropriate for their use at National level.

Monotype, (1977) conducted a study on grip and arm strength in males and females. More than 6,000 males and females aged 10 to 69 in a total community in Tecumseh and Michigan, were given grip and arm strength tests. The eighty two per cent of the entire community who were in that age range are participated in the study. Of this 82 percent, almost all persons without medical contradictions took the strength tests. Percentile scores for both sexes within narrow age ranges were presented. In most populations in which strength had been measured over a wide range, the participants were volunteers; hence it was not possible to define the population. Because of the high participation rate, the Tecumseh sample includes those who ordinarily would volunteer for strength tests, but also those who generally would not. Therefore the percentile scores presented probably represent arm grip strength in healthy males and females than other data which has been published.

Campbell, (1977) designed the Scarborough fitness kit to allow grade nine and ten students to evaluate their level of fitness in seven major areas (agility, flexibility, vital capacity, strength, percentage of body fat, and cardiovascular efficiency) and to provide information that will allow physical education teacher to prescribe a personal fitness programme. Data has been collected from the first year and Scarborough norms for tests selected have been established.

Beckford, (1976) prepared a study to evaluate the physical fitness level of Navajo girls 14, 15 and 16 years old. For AAHPER Youth Fitness Test was administered on the subjects where selected from seven schools of the region to measure the physical fitness level. Also norms were established on basis of sources obtained from test results from these schools. These norms were 60 compared to National Norm were used to this norms found in the manual accompanying the AAHPER Youth Fitness Test. The result of the study gave an indication of the overall fitness level of 14-, 15-, and 16- year old Navajo Girls of the seven test items. The Navajo norms were below the National norms on 5 test items and above on softball throw and 600 yards run and walk.

Callway, (1976) constructed a percentile norm for Albarna students in grade 1-9. These percentile norms were based on both AAPHER youth fitness test. The subjects were 2545 Albarna boys and girls. Norms were constructed for each item based on age and sex. The obtained mean performance on each test items were evaluated by compared with National norms.

Box, (1973) conducted percentile norm tables for selected measures of strength, power, agility, flexibility, body composition, cardiovascular and muscular endurance from data which is collected in five schools of the Unity Christian School System of Hudsonville.

Shore, (1972) constructed motor fitness test battery for lower elementary grade boys. Thirty Experimental test items considered as valid and reliable means uses of motor fitness were administered to 238 boys. After analyzing the data two test batteries containing seven items each were developed on the basis of the rotated factor loading of the test items. Test battery-I contained the highest loaded test item for each factor such as Clark's strength composite; Mc Cloy's endurance ratio; Well's Sit and Reach test; Bass balance or stick; Log flexior can extensor flexibility; Arm flexior or the back flexibility and Modified push-ups test. The second battery-II contained more administratively feasible test items strength such as Grip strength; 300 yard run; Well's sit and reach; Bass balance on stick length wise; Leg flexior and extensor flexibility; Arm flexior or the back flexibility; and modified push ups.

Kinney, (1972) constructed motor fitness test battery for under graduate male physical education Majors. Forty nine test items were selected as valid measures of the eight motor fitness components and were administered to 121 under graduate males. The data were analyzed according to the principle axes method with varimare criterion for rotation. Five factors were isolated and named, speed endurance, gross strength, power, flexibility and relative muscular strength, muscular endurance. Two test batteries having five items each were developed or the basis of the rotated factor loading Test battery I contained highest loading items (1) Time limit shuttle run (2) Cable tension (3) 10-yard dash. (4) Thigh flexor flexibility (5) Bar push-ups. A physical ability test battery for New Zealand schools was developed by modifying the Fleishman battery of physical ability tests by Mc Caughan to produce national norms for a battery of physical ability tests that can be used to assess the relative fitness of New Zealand secondary school boys. Modifying four original test (No. 1, 4, 6 and 9) nine tests recommended by Fleishman were used. Percentile and T-score norms was produced from over 58,000 test scores with the results covering boys of ages 13 to 17 years, in nine tests of physical ability.

Mood, (1971) conducted a study of two forms of the test of physical fitness, knowledge of senior physical education for major students. One hundred and eighty four experimental test items, the contents of which were based on 60 physical fitness facts secured from recent physical education literature and on the opinions of 73 members of the Research Council of AAHPER, were administered to 1,360 physical education major students enrolled in 35 collegiate institutions in the United States. As a result of item analysis data, two parallel forms of the tests were constructed. For the purpose of obtaining validity and reliability of data and establishing national norms the two final test forms were administered to 4,167 students enrolled in 150 collegiate institutions in the United States. Two forms of the test of physical fitness knowledge were constructed so that growth in comparison of physical fitness can be analyzed.

2.3 CRITICAL EVALUATION OF RELATED REVIEWS

The researcher has thoroughly examined the above selected literature, articles and research papers and found that the reviews mentioned above are closely related to the topic selected by the researcher. Though the nature of the researcher conducted earlier by the eminent scholars are slightly different. They are more focused on District of Maharashtra. It has been also observed that no studies have been conducted in order to determine the norms for secondary School Students by any other researcher. The researcher has taken into account the selected variables for studies are not touched. The selected literature helps the researcher to formulate the hypothesis and also to follow the research methodology used in the various researchers in their study.

While critically evaluating the related literature, it also observed by the scholar that various normative studies are available on the Health Related Physical Fitness variables. Since the test, measurement and evaluation concepts developed in Physical Education, there are no specific studies available in order to see the development of norms for Motor Fitness Components for secondary school students of District of Maharashtra. Even though it is the part of their curriculum. Hence, by taking in to consideration the urgent need of developing such Motor Fitness norms, it was thought appropriate by the researcher to undertake the present study.

CHAPTER III

CHAPTER – III

METHODS & MATERIALS

This is a Normative Study, which has a base in Descriptive Research. The purpose of the present study is to develop standard norms of "Health Related Physical Fitness Variable" **for the** Secondary Students of International Schools of Greater Mumbai Aged 11 to 13 years.

3.1 DESIGN OF STUDY

The research design followed, here, a Survey-cum-normative research. This piece of research was conducted to establish **State-wide norms** of Health Related Physical Fitness Test for the school students studying at standards VII (age: 13+ yrs.) and VIII (age: 14+ yrs.) IX (age: 15+ yrs.) in Maharashtra. Standard procedure was employed for this study.

3.2 SELECTION OF POPULATION AND SAMPLE

Considering the stratified random sampling, maximum **3,840 students (i.e., 1,920 boys and 1,920 girls)** from all the educational divisions of Maharashtra state attended for data collection. The subjects' age was ranged from 13 to 15 years, which was decided as per school record. To obtain a representative sample from all over Maharashtra state and to make the study more authentic and reliable, the present investigator chalked out a list of secondary schools to locate the region-wise data. There are eight educational zones in Maharashtra viz., *Nasik, Mumbai, Pune, Kolhapur, Aurangabad, Latur, Nagpur, and Amravati.* The researcher has attended all the said eight educational zones for sampling.

However, the blue print of subjects' distribution has been presented in Table 3.1.

Table 3.1 Blue Print of Sampling

	SUBJECTS												TOTAL
	13 YEARS				14 YEARS				15 YEARS				
	Boys (2 school each)		Girls (2 school each)		Boys (2 school each)		Girls (2 school each)		Boys (2 school each)		Girls (2 school each)		
A	R	U	R	U	R	U	R	U	R	U	R	U	480
	20+ 20	20+ 20	20+ 20	20+ 20	20+ 20	20+ 20	20+ 20	20+ 20	20+ 20	20+ 20	20+ 20	20+ 20	
	80		80		80		80		80		80		
B	R	U	R	U	R	U	R	U	R	U	R	U	480
	20+ 20	20+ 20	20+ 20	20+ 20	20+ 20	20+ 20	20+ 20	20+ 20	20+ 20	20+ 20	20+ 20	20+ 20	
	80		80		80		80		80		80		
C	R	U	R	U	R	U	R	U	R	U	R	U	480
	20+ 20	20+ 20	20+ 20	20+ 20	20+ 20	20+ 20	20+ 20	20+ 20	20+ 20	20+ 20	20+ 20	20+ 20	
	80		80		80		80		80		80		
D	R	U	R	U	R	U	R	U	R	U	R	U	480
	20+ 20	20+ 20	20+ 20	20+ 20	20+ 20	20+ 20	20+ 20	20+ 20	20+ 20	20+ 20	20+ 20	20+ 20	
	80		80		80		80		80		80		
E	R	U	R	U	R	U	R	U	R	U	R	U	480
	20+ 20	20+ 20	20+ 20	20+ 20	20+ 20	20+ 20	20+ 20	20+ 20	20+ 20	20+ 20	20+ 20	20+ 20	
	80		80		80		80		80		80		
F	R	U	R	U	R	U	R	U	R	U	R	U	480
	20+ 20	20+ 20	20+ 20	20+ 20	20+ 20	20+ 20	20+ 20	20+ 20	20+ 20	20+ 20	20+ 20	20+ 20	
	80		80		80		80		80		80		
D	R	U	R	U	R	U	R	U	R	U	R	U	480
	20+ 20	20+ 20	20+ 20	20+ 20	20+ 20	20+ 20	20+ 20	20+ 20	20+ 20	20+ 20	20+ 20	20+ 20	
	80		80		80		80		80		80		
H	R	U	R	U	R	U	R	U	R	U	R	U	480
	20+ 20	20+ 20	20+ 20	20+ 20	20+ 20	20+ 20	20+ 20	20+ 20	20+ 20	20+ 20	20+ 20	20+ 20	
	80		80		80		80		80		80		

3.3 SELECTION OF VARIABLES AND TEST

- The AAHPERD Health Related Physical Fitness Test which was developed in 1980 will be considered as the main tool for this study. It consists of the following components.

Morphological Test	Recommended Test Items
Date of Birth	As per school record
Height	Standing height
Weight	Body weight

- Although many variables of Health Related Physical Fitness, based on various reports as mentioned in the review chapter, were taken into consideration, following variables were finally selected:

Table 3.2
Event wise Test Items

Sr.	**Fitness Components**	**Recommended Test Items**	**Tools Used & Criterion Measures**
1	Abdominal Muscles strength	***Bent Knee Sit Ups***	Stop watch (nearest to 1.0 No. /min.)
2	Muscular Strength	***Push Ups***	Stop watch (nearest to 1.0 No. /min.)
3	Cardio respiratory endurance	**Run / Walk for 9-minute**	Measuring tape & stop watch (Distance covered in 9 minutes was assessed nearest to 0.05 Cm.)
4	Flexibility	**Sit & Reach test**	Cureton's Flexibility box (nearest to 0.05 Cm.)
5	Body Composition	**Skin Fold Measurement**	Skin fold caliber

3.4 DESCRIPTION OF TESTS

3.4.1 BENT KNEE SIT UP

Purpose

To measure abdominal strength and endurance.

Facilities and equipment

Mats be used if they are available, otherwise the floor is satisfactory. Stop watch.

Procedure

The student lies flat on the back with knees bent and feet on the floor with the feet not more than 1 foot from the buttocks. The knee angle should be no less than 90 degrees. The fingers are interlocked and placed behind the neck with the elbows touching the floor. The feet are held securely by a partner the subject then curls up to a sitting position and touch the elbows to knees. This exercise is repeated as many times as possible in the time requirement.

Instruction

Your fingers must remain interlocked and in contact with the back of your neck at all times. You may not push off the floor with an elbow. When you return to the starting position your elbows must be flat on the mat.

Scoring

One point is scored for each correct sit up. The score is maximum number of sit ups completed in 60 seconds.

3.4.2 PUSH UPS TEST

Purpose: To measure strength of upper limbs and shoulder girdle.

Facilities and Equipments: Stopwatch.

Procedure: From prone body position, whole body is lifted upward with the help of hands (palm facing downward) and toes to a balance position At the signal ready!, the subjects make the body very stiff like a wood and then the body comes down by folding the hands at elbow and when nose touches the ground the body is lifted to original position. Thus one count is completed. Likewise the number of counts completed in per minute is recorded as data.

Score: Number of push up completed in one minute is the score.

3.4.3 MINUTE RUN-WALK TEST

Purpose: To measure Cardio-vascular Endurance.

Facilities and Equipment's: Track or marked area and stopwatch.

Procedure: At the signal ready Go!, the subject cover the as much distance as possible in 9 minutes. The tester count the number of laps completed and additional incomplete lap distance covered in 9 minutes.

Score: Cover distance in 9 minutes was count in meter.

Instruction: Subjects can take standing start while running, walking is also permitted but the performer has to cover the distance in 9 minutes.

3.4.4 SIT AND REACH TEST

(Modified - as per Maharashtra State Secondary and Higher Secondary Education Bureau, Pune. GR. No. R.M./PPA/7576 dated 24/10/2007)

Purpose: To evaluate the flexibility of the lower back and posterior thigh.

Instruction: The student assumes a sitting position with legs extended, feet shoulder-width apart and shoes off. The arms are extended forward with one hand on top of the other and finger pads on top of fingernails. The player reaches directly forward, palms down, along the measuring scale four times, holding the position of maximum reach the last time for one full second. Only one trial is given.

Equipment: A level floor or smooth surface ground, a special apparatus consisting of a box with a measuring scale in which 39 cms., is at the edge against which the bottom of the feet rest, score cards or recording sheets, pencil and whistle.

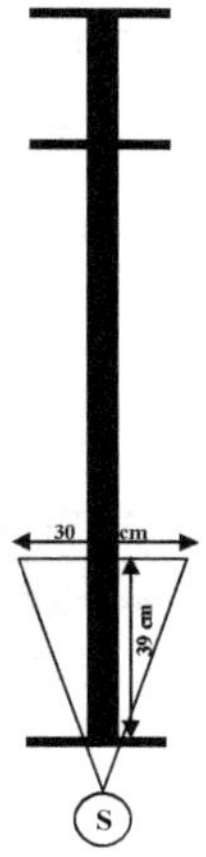

Procedure: Leg must remain straight throughout the entire stretch. The test administrator may need to hold the legs down at the knees. Players take the test with their shoes off. Players can be thought to administer the test to one another. Players should warm up prior to the test. The test apparatus should be placed against the wall to prevent it from sliding on the floor.

Scoring: The score is the most distant point reached, measured toe the nearest centimeter.

3.4.5 Skin Fold Measurement

Purpose

To measure Fat

Facilities and Equipment

Skins fold Caliber, pen or marker

Testing Point

a) Biceps Skinfold Width

b) Triceps Skinfold Width

c) Subscapular Skinfold Width

d) Supra-iliac Skinfold Width

a) Biceps Skinfold Width

Procedure

The subject with a naked arm is asked to stand at ease with hanging arms.Usually, the mid-point of the upper-arm marked previously for measuring upper-arm circumference helps to provide a landmark for measuring biceps and triceps skinfolds as these are also be taken at exactly the same level where the upper-arm circumference is measured. The skin and subcutaneous fat fold is picked at about 1cm above the marked level on the anterior side of the biceps muscle. The jaws of the caliper are applied on the fold so that the marked horizontal line is approximately at a level of the mid-point of the jaws and that the jaws hold a double layer of skin plus subcutaneous fat. The lighter arm of caliper is slowly released so as to put full pressure of the jaws on the vertical skinfold.

b) Triceps Skinfold Width

Procedure

The subject with a naked arm is asked to stand at ease with hanging arms. Usually, the Posterior side of the upper-arm marked previously for measuring Posteriorside of upper-arm circumference helps to provide a landmark for measuring biceps and triceps skinfolds as these are also to be taken at exactly the same level where the Posterior side of upper-arm circumference is measured. The skin and subcutaneous fat fold is picked at about 1cm above the marked level on the Posterior side of the biceps muscle. The jaws of the caliper are applied on the fold so that the marked horizontal line is approximately at a level of the mid-point of the jaws and that the jaws hold a double layer of skin plus subcutaneous fat. The lighter arm of caliper is slowly released so as to put full pressure of the jaws on the vertical skinfold.

c) Subscapular Skinfold Width

Procedure

The skinfold is picked diagonally below the inferior angle of the scapula almost parallel to the medial border of scapula, in such a way that the skinfold forms an angle of roughly $45^0$to the horizontal, with its lower end pointing outwards. The jaws of caliper are applied about half a centimeter below the fold picking tip of the thump. The measurement, as usual, is recorded after two seconds of releasing full pressure on the fold.

d) Supra-illac Skinfold Width

Procedure

A Skinfold is lifted about 1 centimeter above and 2cm medical to the anterior illac spine on the left or Right side. The jaws of the skinfold caliber applied parallel to the natural direction of the picked up skinfold which is usually horizontal or slightly oblique pointing upwards latterly and downwards medially.

Scoring

The reading is noted from the dial of the caliber when the reading quite stable. The measurement is recorded correct up to 0.2 mm.

3.5 METHODS OF ESTABLISHING NORMS

The procedure of standardization and development of norms of **Health Related Physical Fitness Test'** was be followed by ***two stages***:

- ***Stage I:*** involves formation of test-items, determination of content validity, first try-out, and second try-out to get a '*preliminary form*' of developing Norms.
- ***Stage II:*** includes establishment of final norms, test's reliability and validity.

Stage I

- This stage involves the determination of content validity, first try-out, and second try-out to get a '*preliminary form*' of developing Norms.
- The technique, design and strategy for construction as well as evaluation of each item were formulated and improved. Each of the formulated fitness ability can be called as **'test-item'**. The preliminary value of **content validity** was assessed by considering the judgement of various experts in the area of Physical Education and Sports and on the basis of investigator's professional experience. The number of newly formulated test-items was then modified to include in the **'Health Related Physical Fitness Test'**.
- Minimum two hundred (n=200 i.e., boys and girls) school students, age ranging from each age group, from schools of urban and sub-urban of Ahmed Nagar area were tested primarily by administering the tests on **'first try-out'** basis. The detailed distribution of the subjects has been presented in Chapter IV. The Split half reliability coefficient was assessed for each test-item and also for the test as a whole. The significant reliability coefficient ensured the **'Preliminary Form'** of the test (Chapter IV).

Stage II

In the 'final stage', each item was arranged systematically by following 'simple to complex' order. The **'time limit'** for performing each test-item of the Physical Fitness Test was recorded. The **'norms'** of the said test were established. The **'content validity'** of the test was established. The **Split-half reliability** coefficient of both the tests was determined. This, in fact, ensured the '**Final Form**' of the '**Physical Fitness Test**'.

3.6 RELIABILITY AND VALIDITY OF THE INSTRUMENTS USED FOR TESTING

Reliability of data was ensured by establishing reliability of tests, reliability of tools and tester's competency as given below.

3.8.1 Reliability of Tests

Although the reliability and validity coefficients of each test item have been presented in Chapter IV, the result revealed that test items were found reliable at the 0.01 level.

3.8.2 Reliability of Tools

The tools such as stopwatches, measuring tape, sit and reach box, etc. used in testing are standardized.

The steel tape was used for measuring the distance in 9min-run-walk, whereas Sit and Reach box was used to measure flexibility.

Since the measuring tape and sit and reach box were non-elastic (supplied by Freemans, India) and stop watches were electronic (supplied by Seiko Company), it is assumed that the instruments used were reliable.

All the instruments used were taken from the Research Laboratory of Bombay Physical Culture Association's College of Physical Education, Wadala,Mumbai-31. All the tools were tested before their use in testing and found functioning.

3.8.3 Testers' Competency

All the measurements were taken by the present researcher himself with the assistance of some other professionally qualified staff members working in the BPCA's College of Physical Education, Mumbai.

Before going for the original data collection, the scholar had a number of practice sessions along with assistants.

To establish the testers' competency, ten subjects were chosen at random and tests were taken on them by the research scholar and the assistants under identical conditions. The reliability coefficients were found to be within the range of 0.86 to 0.94.

3.7 STATISTICAL TECHNIQUES USED

The data were analysed using the following statistical techniques:

- The reliability of the Preliminary form of the test was determined by **split-half method** of correlation.
- Content validity was determined by analysing the opinions of the various experts in the area of education and physical education.
- Before establishing the norms, the distribution of performance scores of each item of physical fitness test were assessed with respect to a normal probability curve. Here, normality of the scores was evaluated on the basis of the values of Kolmogorov-Smirnova Test of Normality.
- After **testing the normality** of the item-wise performance scores of the subjects, the data were processed for calculation of Percentile norms.
- The item-wise normative data were **graded** on the basis of the principles of Likert's Five point scale (Guilford & Fruchter, 1973).

CHAPTER IV

CHAPTER IV

ANALYSIS AND INTERPRETATION

As per the research design, the details of data analysis and interpretation of results have been presented in this chapter.

4.1 RESULTS ON DEVELOPMENT OF NORMS OF PHYSICAL FITNESS TEST

It has been stated in the earlier chapter that the technique of development of norms considers three stages:

- Stage I
- Stage II

The results obtained in each stage have been presented below:

4.1.1 RESULT ON STAGE I (First Try-Out)

On the basis of recommendation and results of earlier report (Pargaonkar, 2002, Jadhav, 2014 and Aher, 2016) following test-items of Physical Fitness test have been identified:

- Muscular Endurance
- Muscular Strength
- Cardio-Vascular Endurance
- Flexibility
- Body Composititon

These test items were administered on 13 Years Boys (n1=320) & Girls (n1=320), 14 Years Boys (n1=320) & Girls (n1=320) and 15 Years Boys (n1=320) & Girls (n1=320) who were randomly assigned with the help of Fisher's random table, on try-out basis from urban and sub-urban areas in Greater Mumbai (Maharashtra) (Table 4.1).

Table 4.1:

Gender wise and Age wise Sample

	SUBJECTS												**TOTAL**
	13 YEARS				**14 YEARS**				**15 YEARS**				
	Boys (2 school each)		**Girls (2 school each)**		**Boys (2 school each)**		**Girls (2 school each)**		**Boys (2 school each)**		**Girls (2 school each)**		
A	R	U	R	U	R	U	R	U	R	U	R	U	480
	20+ 20	20+ 20	20+ 20	20+ 20	20+ 20	20+ 20	20+ 20	20+ 20	20+ 20	20+ 20	20+ 20	20+ 20	
	80		80		80		80		80		80		
B	R	U	R	U	R	U	R	U	R	U	R	U	480
	20+ 20	20+ 20	20+ 20	20+ 20	20+ 20	20+ 20	20+ 20	20+ 20	20+ 20	20+ 20	20+ 20	20+ 20	
	80		80		80		80		80		80		
C	R	U	R	U	R	U	R	U	R	U	R	U	480
	20+ 20	20+ 20	20+ 20	20+ 20	20+ 20	20+ 20	20+ 20	20+ 20	20+ 20	20+ 20	20+ 20	20+ 20	
	80		80		80		80		80		80		
D	R	U	R	U	R	U	R	U	R	U	R	U	480
	20+ 20	20+ 20	20+ 20	20+ 20	20+ 20	20+ 20	20+ 20	20+ 20	20+ 20	20+ 20	20+ 20	20+ 20	
	80		80		80		80		80		80		
E	R	U	R	U	R	U	R	U	R	U	R	U	480
	20+ 20	20+ 20	20+ 20	20+ 20	20+ 20	20+ 20	20+ 20	20+ 20	20+ 20	20+ 20	20+ 20	20+ 20	
	80		80		80		80		80		80		
F	R	U	R	U	R	U	R	U	R	U	R	U	480
	20+ 20	20+ 20	20+ 20	20+ 20	20+ 20	20+ 20	20+ 20	20+ 20	20+ 20	20+ 20	20+ 20	20+ 20	
	80		80		80		80		80		80		
D	R	U	R	U	R	U	R	U	R	U	R	U	480
	20+ 20	20+ 20	20+ 20	20+ 20	20+ 20	20+ 20	20+ 20	20+ 20	20+ 20	20+ 20	20+ 20	20+ 20	
	80		80		80		80		80		80		
H	R	U	R	U	R	U	R	U	R	U	R	U	480
	20+ 20	20+ 20	20+ 20	20+ 20	20+ 20	20+ 20	20+ 20	20+ 20	20+ 20	20+ 20	20+ 20	20+ 20	
	80		80		80		80		80		80		

4.1.2 RESULTS ON NORMALITY OF DATA

It is a common procedure that establishing the norms of a test is possible only if the related data are representing a mostly normal probability curve. Therefore, the normality of distribution of scores as obtained from each test of the Health Related Physical Fitness was statistically tested separately with the help of Shapiro-W Kolmogorov-Smirnova test. After finding out the nature of distribution and on the basis of the characteristics of probability curve, the percentile norms each test item were determined.

Table 4.2:

Kolmogorov-Smirnov and Shapiro-Wilk Test of Normality of Health Related Physical Fitness of Male Students of Age 13 Years

	Kolmogorov-Smirnov			Shapiro-Wilk		
	Statistic	**df**	**Sig.**	**Statistic**	**df**	**Sig.**
Muscular Endurance	0.091	40	0.200	0.963	40	0.208
Muscular Strength	0.069	40	0.200	0.970	40	0.354
Cardiovascular Endurance	0.126	40	0.109	0.965	40	0.249
Flexibility	0.145	40	0.134	0.951	40	0.184
Body Composition	0.135	40	0.164	0.911	40	0.104

Table 4.3:

Kolmogorov-Smirnov and Shapiro-Wilk Test of Normality of Health Related Physical Fitness of Female Students of Age 13 Years

	Kolmogorov-Smirnov			Shapiro-Wilk		
	Statistic	**df**	**Sig.**	**Statistic**	**df**	**Sig.**
Muscular Endurance	0.09	41	0.200	0.982	41	0.737
Muscular Strength	0.118	41	0.168	0.975	41	0.482
Cardiovascular Endurance	0.107	41	0.200	0.973	41	0.416
Flexibility	0.145	41	0.031	0.959	41	0.145
Body Composition	0.109	41	0.100	0.781	41	0.638

From table 4.2 and 4.3 the scores of Health Related Physical Fitness were normally distributed, as assessed by Kolmogorov-Smirnova test for large group ($p > .05$). It can, therefore, be said that the distribution of scores of Health Related Physical Fitness is nearly normal in Male and Female Students.

4.1.3 RESULTS ON RELIABILITY OF DATA

Split-half reliability test was used to establish to reliability coefficients of the 'Preliminary form' of the tests. For this the scores of each item of each group were split into two halves. The first half contained performance score of odd numbered students and the second half contained even numbered student. The coefficients of split-half reliability of each item for boys and girls have been presented in Tables 4.3.

Table 4.4:

Reliability Coefficients of the Items of the Preliminary Form of the Physical Fitness Test for the School Students Ages 13 to 15 Years

Reliability and Validity of tools			
Code No. of Item	**Variables**	**Reliability**	**Validity**
	Fitness dimensions		
A1	CV Endurance	0.99	0.99
A2	Muscular strength	0.83	0.66
A3	Muscular endurance	0.95	0.92
A4	Flexibility	0.99	0.99
A5	Speed	0.95	0.88

The result of split-half reliability in Tables 4.2 indicates that the reliability coefficient of the items viz., Push Ups (A1), Sit ups Test (A2), 9 mts run and Walk (A3), Sit and Reach Test (A4) and Body Composition (A5), in the newly formed Tests 0.99, 0.83, 0.95, 0.99 and 0.95 respectively, and Validity coefficient was 0.99, 0.66, 0.92, 0.99 and 0.88. It is amazing to note that the reliability and validity coefficients for all selected Variables were statistically significant.

Since the test-items of Physical fitness were authenticated by several experts in physical education and sports sciences and are used by the teachers of physical education, the items bear face validity.

4.2 RESULT ON STAGE II (ESTABLISHING NORMS)

4.2.1 RESULTS ON ESTABLISHING NORMS OF MALE STUDENTS

4.2.1 RESULTS ON PERCENTILE OF MUSCULAR ENDURANCE

Table 4.5:

Percentile of Muscular Endurance Variables of Male Students belonging to age of 13, 14 and 15 Years

Muscular Endurance				
Age		13 Year	14 Year	15 Year
Percentiles	10	22.00	22. 50	16.00
	20	23.50	24.60	20.50
	30	24.33	25.86	24.00
	40	25.00	28.50	26.75
	50	26.78	33.00	29.14
	60	29.00	34.46	31.20
	70	30.25	35.17	35.33
	80	32.50	35.83	37.86
	90	33.00	38.67	40.50
	100	36.00	40.00	44.00

The result of percentile norms indicates that the P10 and P100 values of the Muscular Endurance were "36 & above" and "22 & below" for 13 Years, "40 & above" and "22.50 & below" for 14 Years and "44 & above" and "16 & below" for 15 Years respectively.

4.2.1.2 RESULTS ON PERCENTILE OF MUSCULAR STRENGTH

Table 4.6:

Percentile of Muscular Strength Variables of Male Students belonging to age of 13, 14 and 15 Years

Muscular Strength				
Age		13 Year	14 Year	15 Year
Perc	10	17.33	17.25	19.50
	20	18.67	19.17	21.33

	30	20.17	20.60	23.15
	40	21.75	23.00	24.25
	50	23.50	25.33	25.67
	60	24.63	26.67	27.00
	70	25.63	28.00	28.25
	80	27.00	29.50	30.00
	90	30.50	30.57	31.00
	100	32.00	32.500	32.67

The result of percentile norms indicates that the P10 and P100 values of the Muscular Strength were "32 & above" and "17.33 & below" for 13 Years, "32.50 & above" and "17.25 & below" for 14 Years and "32.67 & above" and "19.50 & below" for 15 Years respectively.

4.2.1.3 RESULTS ON PERCENTILE OF CARDIOVASCULAR ENDURANCE

Table 4.7

Percentile of Cardiovascular Endurance Variables of Male Students belonging to age of 13, 14 and 15 Years

Cardiovascular Endurance				
Age		13 Year	14 Year	15 Year
Percentiles	10	1175.00	1360.00	1362.50
	20	1272.50	1503.00	1457.50
	30	1306.67	1537.50	1528.75
	40	1346.25	1625.00	1565.00
	50	1402.50	1655.00	1656.67
	60	1443.75	1703.33	1710.00
	70	1537.50	1740.00	1770.00
	80	1595.00	1820.00	1860.00
	90	1693.33	1853.33	1905.00
	100	1880.00	1950.00	19560.00

The result of percentile norms indicates that the P10 and P100 values of the Cardiovascular Endurance were "1880 & above" and "1175 & below" for 13 Years, "1950

& above" and "1360& below" for 14 Years and "19560& above" and "1362 & below" for 15 Years respectively.

4.2.1.4 RESULTS ON PERCENTILE OF FLEXIBILITY

Table 4.8

Percentile of Flexibility Variables of Male Students belonging to age of 13, 14 and 15 Years

Flexibility				
Age		13 Year	14 Year	15 Year
Percentiles	10	21.00	25.00	26.40
	20	26.00	28.67	28.80
	30	29.20	29.75	30.08
	40	30.80	31.20	30.75
	50	31.88	33.60	31.46
	60	32.88	35.33	32.33
	70	34.25	37.60	33.80
	80	36.50	39.50	35.67
	90	38.00	41.50	39.00
	100	42.00	42.50	47.00

The result of percentile norms indicates that the P10 and P100 values of the Flexibility were "42& above" and "21 & below" for 13 Years, "42.50 & above" and "25 & below" for 14 Years and "47 & above" and "26.40 & below" for 15 Years respectively.

4.2.1.5 RESULTS ON PERCENTILE OF BODY COMPOSITION

Table 4.9

Percentile of Body Composition Variables of Male Students belonging to age of 13, 14 and 15 Years

Body Composition				
Age		13 Year	14 Year	15 Year
Percentiles	10	08.91	09.14	11.08
	20	10.32	10.24	12.15
	30	12.45	11.72	12.77
	40	14.57	12.89	13.78

	50	15.48	13.74	14.35
	60	16.08	14.33	14.78
	70	16.56	14.86	15.38
	80	17.20	15.64	16.69
	90	18.59	18.13	18.39
	100	20.98	22.00	22.35

The result of percentile norms indicates that the P10 and P100 values of the Body Composition were "20.98 & above" and "08.91 & below" for 13 Years, "22 & above" and "09.14 & below" for 14 Years and "22.35 & above" and "11.08 & below" for 15 Years respectively.

4.2.2 RESULTS ON ESTABLISHING NORMS OF FEMALE STUDENTS

4.2.2.1 RESULTS ON PERCENTILE OF MUSCULAR ENDURANCE

Table 4.10

Percentile of Muscular Endurance Variables of Female Students belonging to age of 13, 14 and 15 Years

Muscular Endurance				
Age		**13 Year**	**14 Year**	**15 Year**
Percentiles	**10**	15.25	16.25	16.47
	20	20.28	18.50	17.50
	30	21.92	21.67	19.43
	40	23.35	24.20	20.57
	50	24.50	25.80	23.50
	60	25.87	30.75	28.50
	70	27.20	34.50	35.40
	80	28.43	37.33	39.00
	90	29.90	40.00	41.00
	100	31.60	42.00	42.10

The result of percentile norms indicates that the P10 and P100 values of the Muscular Endurance were "31.60 & above" and "15.25 & below" for 13 Years, "42.00 & above" and "16.25 & below" for 14 Years and "42.10 & above" and "16.47 & below" for 15 Years respectively.

4.2.2.2 RESULTS ON PERCENTILE OF MUSCULAR STRENGTH

Table 4.11

Percentile of Muscular Strength Variables of Female Students belonging to age of 13, 14 and 15 Years

Muscular Strength				
Age		13 Year	14 Year	15 Year
Percentiles	10	15.44	15.57	19.73
	20	17.17	24.31	21.00
	30	18.75	25.83	30.00
	40	22.00	28.12	35.83
	50	24.50	30.00	41.50
	60	26.88	31.64	46.33
	70	30.00	33.08	48.20
	80	34.00	35.80	50.00
	90	36.05	37.00	52.00
	100	38.40	40.80	53.00

The result of percentile norms indicates that the P10 and P100 values of the Muscular Strength were "38.40 & above" and "15.44 & below" for 13 Years, "40.80 & above" and "15.57 & below" for 14 Years and "53 & above" and "19.73 & below" for 15 Years respectively.

4.2.2.3 RESULTS ON PERCENTILE OF CARDIOVASCULAR ENDURANCE

Table 4.12

Percentile of Cardiovascular Endurance Variables of Female Students belonging to age of 13, 14 and 15 Years

Cardiovascular Endurance				
Age		13 Year	14 Year	15 Year
Percentiles	10	1055.00	1264.00	1267.50
	20	1086.67	1348.50	1295.00
	30	1153.75	1367.67	1312.00
	40	1250.00	1386.00	1330.00
	50	1300.00	1430.00	1347.50
	60	1335.00	1471.50	1375.00
	70	1380.00	1571.00	1443.33
	80	1426.67	1591.50	1485.00
	90	1490.00	1628.00	1570.00
	100	1590.00	1650.00	1660.00

The result of percentile norms indicates that the P10 and P100 values of the Cardiovascular Endurance were "1590 & above" and "1055 & below" for 12 Years, "1650 & above" and "1264 & below" for 14 Years and "1660 & above" and "1267 & below" for 15 Years respectively.

4.2.2.4 RESULTS ON PERCENTILE OF FLEXIBILITY

Table 4.13

Percentile of Flexibility Variables of Female Students belonging to age of 13, 14 and 15 Years

Flexibility				
Age		13 Year	14 Year	15 Year
Percenti	10	21.50	21.96	26.50
	20	29.00	25.73	29.20
	30	32.75	28.20	30.00

	40	33.88	30.22	30.73
	50	35.33	30.85	32.00
	60	37.75	34.06	34.00
	70	39.33	36.40	36.33
	80	40.67	39.20	39.67
	90	42.80	41.00	42.00
	100	43.00	43.80	45.50

The result of percentile norms indicates that the P10 and P100 values of the Flexibility were "43 & above" and "21.50 & below" for 13 Years, "43.80 & above" and "21.96 & below" for 14 Years and "45.50 & above" and "26.50 & below" for 15 Years respectively.

4.2.2.5 RESULTS ON PERCENTILE OF BODY COMPOSITION

Table 4.14

Percentile of Body Composition Variables of Female Students belonging to age of 13, 14 and 15 Years

Body Composition				
Age		13 Year	14 Year	15 Year
Percentiles	10	10.85	13.36	16.87
	20	12.91	16.43	17.62
	30	13.86	17.58	18.44
	40	15.10	18.67	19.42
	50	16.21	19.51	20.32
	60	16.87	21.30	21.45
	70	17.75	21.81	21.80
	80	18.75	22.50	22.12
	90	20.71	23.73	22.96
	100	22.20	24.03	24.61

The result of percentile norms indicates that the P10 and P100 values of the Body Composition were "22.20 & above" and "10.85 & below" for 13 Years, "24.03 & above" and "13.36 & below" for 14 Years and "24.61 & above" and "16.87 & below" for 15 Years respectively.

4.3 RESULTS ON DERIVATION OF GRADES IN HEALTH RELATED PHYSICAL FITNESS TEST OF MALE STUDENTS

The results of the percentile norms presented above were further substantiated to find out grade in the performance in the Health Related Physical Fitness Test for Male Students. The grade of raw scores in each test-item can be identified on the basis of Likert's Five points scale. The raw score achieved in each event can be well interpreted easily so that an individual's performance in each event is either excellent or good or average or fair or poor can easily be determined. They have been presented in **Tables 4.16, 4.17 and 4.18.**

Table 4.15

Grading Norms of Health Related Physical Fitness Variables of Male Students belonging to age of 13 Years

		Muscular Endurance	Muscular Strength	Cardiovascular Endurance	Flexibility	Body Composition
Norms	Poor	24	19	1213.33	25.00	11.50
	Fair	26	25	1301.67	29.67	14.81
	Average	29	27	1370.00	30.00	15.96
	Good	32	29	1433.33	32.67	16.87
	Excellent	36	34	1570.00	39.00	18.96

Table 4.16

Grading Norms of Health Related Physical Fitness Variables of Male Students belonging to age of 14 Years

		Muscular Endurance	Muscular Strength	Cardiovascular Endurance	Flexibility	Body Composition
Nor	Poor	25	23	1315.00	22.50	10.82
	Fair	30	27	1376.67	29.00	13.16

	Average	35	31	1475.00	30.00	14.47
	Good	38	40	1561.67	35.00	15.15
	Excellent	43	49	1649.17	39.00	18.58

Table 4.17

Grading Norms of Health Related Physical Fitness Variables of Male Students belonging to age of 15 Years

		Muscular Endurance	Muscular Strength	Cardiovascular Endurance	Flexibility	Body Composition
Norms	Poor	22	20	1229.17	22.83	12.67
	Fair	27	25	1360.00	29.00	13.93
	Average	32	28	1397.50	33.00	14.73
	Good	36	32	1495.00	40.00	16.27
	Excellent	41	37	1653.33	42.00	20.38

4.4 RESULTS ON DERIVATION OF GRADES IN HEALTH RELATED PHYSICAL FITNESS TEST OF FEMALE STUDENTS

The results of the percentile norms presented above were further substantiated to find out grade in the performance in the Health Related Physical Fitness Test for Female Students. The grade of raw scores in each test-item can be identified on the basis of Likert's Five points scale. The raw score achieved in each event can be well interpreted easily so that an individual's performance in each event is either excellent or good or average or fair or poor can easily be determined. They have been presented in **Tables 4.19, 4.20 and 4.21**.

Table 4.18

Grading Norms of Health Related Physical Fitness Variables of Female Students belonging to age of 13 Years

		Muscular Endurance	Muscular Strength	Cardiovascular Endurance	Flexibility	Body Composition
Norms	Poor	15	20	1350.00	30.00	13.36
	Fair	21	23	1380.00	31.00	15.96
	Average	23	25	1460.00	32.00	16.87

	Good	26	27	1580.00	36.00	18.52
	Excellent	30	34	1670.00	40.00	21.91

Table 4.19

Grading Norms of Health Related Physical Fitness Variables of Female Students belonging to age of 14 Years

		Muscular Endurance	Muscular Strength	Cardiovascular Endurance	Flexibility	Body Composition
Norms	Poor	18	16	1308.33	29.00	18.45
	Fair	21	20	1343.33	31.00	19.63
	Average	25	25	1528.00	32.00	21.61
	Good	30	30	1680.00	34.00	23.42
	Excellent	35	44	1823.33	38.00	25.32

Table 4.20

Grading Norms of Health Related Physical Fitness Variables of Female Students belonging to age of 15 Years

		Muscular Endurance	Muscular Strength	Cardiovascular Endurance	Flexibility	Body Composition
Norms	Poor	17	15	1095.00	30.00	18.06
	Fair	21	18	1313.33	33.67	19.63
	Average	24	21	1505.00	35.00	21.61
	Good	25	25	1683.33	38.00	22.01
	Excellent	30	28	1863.33	39.17	23.42

5.5 MAJOR FINDINGS

- Health Related Physical Fitness were normally distributed, as assessed by Kolmogorov-Smirnova test for large group ($p > .05$). It can, therefore, be said that the distribution of scores of Health Related Physical Fitness is nearly normal.
- The percentile norms of 5 finally selected test items indicate that the distribution of scores of almost all the test-items resides in the normal range of a probability curve.

- The performance norms of each event (item) were graded as poor, fair, average, good, and excellent on the basis of Likert's five-point scale. The findings indicate that the physical fitness of School Children must be evaluated on the basis of following items:
    - Muscular Endurance (as measured by Bent Knee Sit up).
    - Muscular Strength (as determined by Pull Ups).
    - Cardiovascular Endurance (as measured by 9 minutes Run Walk Test).
    - Sit and Reach (as assessed by Sit and Reach test).
    - Body Composition (as measured by Skin Fold Calliper).

4.6 DISCUSSION OF RESULTS

Physical fitness is a challenging concept in human society. It has been accepted that physical fitness leads towards human health. Since it is essential for every human, the children's physical fitness should not be overlooked. Although, every state government in India has given stress on physical education in schools for maintaining physical fitness of school students, research based information towards benefit are lacking. Many state governments have prepared syllabus of physical education for improvement of physical fitness among the school students, however, standard procedure for evaluation of fitness is beyond the reach of physical education teachers. It was, therefore, thought desirable to develop and standardize a norms to assess the physical fitness status of the school students especially for the Maharashtra State.

The present investigator has taken severe pain to locate the sample throughout the Greater Mumbai and to get permission from the school to collect data. He accepted it as a challenge. He painstakingly made few groups of experts for data collection throughout the state. Finally, he was successful in collecting the data required for this study.

The result revealed that the preliminary form of the test consisted of many test-items and all these items were found reliable and the reliability coefficients were accepted at the 0.01 level of confidence. Moreover, the preliminary form of the test was also found valid.

To get more accuracy in construction of the norms in physical fitness, Researcher ensures that the preliminary form of the test was more concise and the test was then administered on the large sample. Prior to establishing the norms, normality of the data on each test item was tested with help of Kolmogorov-Smirnova test. Amazingly, all the data of test items were found normal and then they were processed for establishing the norms.

The hypothesis was further tested regarding the reliability and validity of the new formed test norms. The result revealed that the hypothesis as formulated in the thesis has been retained statistically at the 0.01 level. Thus, the test norms were found reliable and valid to measure the Students physical fitness.

Merely, establishing the norms does not have value until the norms are graded. In this study, the researcher has formulated the grades on the basis of Likert's five-point scale. Now the new test battery as developed and standardized in this study got a full form to be administered to assess physical fitness of any children in the age group 11 to 13 years belonging to the Maharashtra State.

CPSIA information can be obtained
at www.ICGtesting.com
Printed in the USA
LVHW080004061222
734629LV00016B/1285

9 789468 492534